D1176831

Fatty Liver

Recipes And Guide To Prevent And Reverse Fatty Liver, Lose Weight And Live Longer

AMY ZACKARY

Copyright © 2017 Amy Zachary

All rights reserved. No part of this publication may be reproduced, distributed, or transmitted in any form or by any means, including photocopying, recording, or other electronic or mechanical methods, without the prior written permission of the publisher, except in the case of brief quotations embodied in critical reviews and certain other noncommercial uses permitted by copyright law.

Limit of Liability/Disclaimer of Warranty: While the publisher and author have used their best efforts in preparing this book, they make no representations or warranties with respect to the accuracy or completeness of the contents of this book and specifically disclaim any implied warranties of merchantability or fitness for a particular purpose. No warranty may be created or extended by sales representatives or written sales materials. The advice and strategies contained herein may not be suitable for your situation. You should consult with a professional where appropriate. Neither the publisher nor author shall be liable for any loss of profit or any other commercial damages, including but not limited to special, incidental, consequential, or other damages.

ISBN-13:978-1978360051

ISBN-10:1978360053

DEDICATION

To those concerned about their health

TABLE OF CONTENTS

Other Books By Amy Zackary

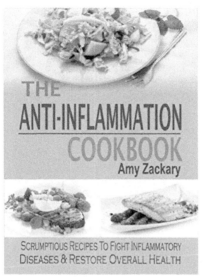

THE ANTI-INFLAMMATION COOKBOOK: SCRUMPTIOUS
RECIPES TO FIGHT INFLAMMATORY DISEASES & RESTORE
OVERALL HEALTH

INTRODUCTION

A healthy liver is imperative to life. If you want to lead a long and healthy life, you must take care of your liver. This large and very important organ supports a large number of other organs in the body. Weighing about 3 pounds in an average adult, the liver performs several essential functions: It detoxifies the blood. It stores nutrients (vitamin and iron) within the body, providing the tissues with the required energy and nutrients. The liver is also a gland because it produces bile, a vital substance for digesting fats.

We all need a healthy liver to survive. A normal, healthy and functioning liver is reddish brown in color. It rids the body of toxin, and helps it to burn excessive fat through the bile. It also helps to maintain a proper weight. On the contrary, a fatty liver is yellow in color, greasy, enlarged and of course, swollen with fat. Instead of helping to burn fat, it stores it. It is also unable to perform many other vital functions. The liver is the body's main detoxifying organ. Nevertheless, it can be destroyed by dangerous toxins in fatty liver.

Fatty liver simply means that there's too much fat in the liver; much more than the liver can process. The result of this is an accumulation of fats in the liver cell, infiltrating the healthy liver areas and putting the liver in great risk. It is normal for the liver to contain some fat. However, if more than 5% to 10% of the liver's total weight is fat, then it is called a fatty liver (steatosis).

Fatty liver is not a disease, but a medical condition that can become a disease as it progresses. This disease affects about one-third of American adults. It is also one of the major causes of liver failure. Fatty liver disease can also cause liver inflammation, permanent liver damage, liver scarring, liver failure and ultimately, death. Fatty liver can also increase your risk of heart attack.

Types Of Fatty Liver

There are two types of fatty liver: Alcohol-related and non-alcohol related.

Alcohol-Related

As the name indicates, alcohol- related fatty liver or alcoholic fatty liver is caused by heavy consumption of alcohol. Generally, excessive alcohol does the liver no good. It diverts it from focusing on its core function of metabolizing carbohydrates and supplying the body with glucose to metabolizing alcohol. By trying to break down alcohol, the liver can bring about some chemical reaction (oxidation) that can damage its cells, resulting in fat deposits. This causes alcohol-induced fatty liver disease. Drinking too much alcohol can result in inflammation (alcoholic hepatitis), and scarring of the liver (cirrhosis).

If, as a man, you are drinking more than 21 units of alcohol in a week, you are drinking too much. For women, drinking more than 14 units of alcohol per week is considered excessive. (One unit is about 10 ml of pure alcohol). If you continue to drink excessive alcohol unchecked for two years and more, you will develop fatty liver.

However, this first stage of injury to your liver can be completely reversed by abstaining from alcohol. But if you have liver disease, even taking the smallest amount of alcohol could worsen your condition. The most important change to make to your diet is to abstain from alcohol or reduce your consumption. You also need to eat a balanced diet, with adequate amount of protein and carbohydrate.

Non -Alcohol Related

Non- alcoholic fatty liver is an accumulation of fat in liver cells that isn't caused by alcohol use. It is a newly diagnosed type of fatty liver, which affects 33 percent Americans, including 6 million children and which is the main focus of this book.

Known as Non-Alcoholic Fatty Liver Disease, (NAFLD), it is a progression from fatty liver and poses a great risk to people who are obese, overweight, who have diabetes and high cholesterol. As a matter of fact, NAFDL is now topping the liver transplant list; not sparing the little ones, as it has been established as the number one liver condition in children. Estimates indicate that about 30 percent of American adult may have fatty liver. This condition can begin as early as childhood. But it is more prevalent in people with type 2 diabetes (about 50 percent) or overweight (about 75 percent). Some people develop NAFLD even if they do not have any risk factors.

It is interesting to note that NAFLD is not caused by eating too much fatty foods, but rather an overconsumption of sugar and processed carbohydrate, since carbs produce more fat in your liver. Besides poor eating habits, another factor that may cause fatty liver is rapid weight loss. Fatty liver is usually associated with abdominal obesity, insulin resistance and type 2 diabetes (the body does not respond normally to insulin). If severe, it can eventually lead to cirrhosis and liver failure.

Symptoms Of Fatty Liver

At the early stages, the symptoms of fatty liver are not noticeable. Many people who have them do not even know that they have a liver problem. As the disorder progresses, the affected individuals may begin to feel unwell, with frequent fatigues or one or two other persistent mild symptoms. However, if the condition advances untreated over a number of years, with no complications, the untreated fatty liver disease will eventually lead to liver failure. This is why you must see a doctor if you have any of these persistent signs and symptoms:

- Nausea
- loss of appetite
- weakness
- Gallstones
- Red itchy eyes
- Spider-like blood vessels
- Overheating of the body
- Jaundice
- Itching
- Edema (swelling of the legs)
- Weight excess in the abdominal area
- Excessive sweating
- mental confusion

So how do you know you have fatty liver? Fatty liver can be diagnosed with blood tests and a liver ultrasound. If your blood test indicates abnormality, then you should start taking steps to reverse. If the blood test indicates normality, you should still do all it takes to prevent it. However, it is best to do a liver ultrasound because it is more sensitive and reliable.

Reversing Fatty Liver

Thankfully, fatty liver is reversible. If you are prone to fatty liver disease, there are several things you can do to prevent it. You can also reduce your risk for fatty liver disease by leading a moderate, healthy lifestyle. Some of these include:

Diet & Nutrition

Good nutrition has been proven to be part of an effective treatment for fatty liver; poor diet being the main cause of fatty liver disease. To reverse it, a good diet with adequate calories, carbohydrates, fats and proteins is essential. This will bring about a regeneration of new liver cells. By eating healthy, the liver will function well, and for a very long time.

People with liver disease must eat a healthy diet to enable the liver function appropriately and help repair some liver damage. If your diet is unhealthy, the liver will work harder to do its job and this can damage it. Therefore, if you are at risk of fatty liver, you should:

Eat Less Carbs

Foods high in carbohydrates have been confirmed to be the major cause of fatty liver since the liver converts excess carbohydrates fats. Avoid sugars and foods that are made of white flour. Limit carbohydrates like white bread, white pasta and pastries. Even whole grain flours should be avoided as it can increase blood sugar levels, stress the liver and result in high triglycerides. This ultimately promotes a fatty liver. Adopt a low carb diet and reduce intake of sugar, especially from candies, crackers and even salad dressing. Eat complex carbs like brown rice, cereals, whole wheat pasta and oatmeal.

Drink Less Alcohol

Of course, you'll have to reduce your intake of alcohol or stop completely. Excess alcohol consumption has been proven to the second major cause of fatty liver. It causes inflammation and damages the liver cells, resulting in fatty liver. If you have fatty liver, it is advisable to limit your alcohol intake to one drink per day and abstain for 2 to 3 days before taking your next one drink.

To avoid fatty liver, men shouldn't drink more than 4 units of alcohol in a day while women shouldn't drink more than 3 units in a day (One unit being about 10 ml of pure alcohol).

Increase Protein Intake

Eat more proteins. Protein helps to stabilize blood sugar levels. It also aids abdominal weight loss as well as reduce hunger and cravings. Ensure protein is taken with each meal, especially breakfast. Eggs, seafood, poultry, meat, seeds, nuts, lentils and beans as well as low-fat dairy products are some good examples of proteins to eat. However, do not eat uncooked shellfish.

Eat The Right Fats

Eat healthy unsaturated fats. Most vegetable oil and margarines can aggravate a fatty liver. Healthy fats intake also help to combat liver damage caused by sugar. Olive oil, nut oil, oily fish, coconut oil, avocados, macadamia, flaxseeds and grass-fed butter should regularly feature in your diet.

Additionally, eat foods that rich in omega 3 fatty acids. You can get this from wild fish, walnuts, and chia and flax seedss.

Eat More Vegetables

Raw vegetables and fruits are very effective for healing the liver and for keeping it in good shape. They cleanse and repair the liver, enabling it to excellently perform its function of removing excess fat and toxins from the blood. Eat lots of vegetables in the form of salads and even cooked ones. While fruits are a healthy consideration, people with high blood sugar or insulin are advised to limit consumption to 2 servings daily.

Cruciferous plants like broccoli and cauliflower are good for the liver. Leafy vegetables like kale, cabbage, collards, watercress and arugula should also be eaten regularly. Garlic is highly effective in detoxifying the body. Onions too, are loaded with sulfur that helps to cleanse the blood. Our liver loves bell peppers, carrots, fresh tomatoes, oranges, lemons, pumpkin and grapefruits. Daily consumption of these vegetables will help to heal and repair the liver.

If you like juicing, then you're in luck! Raw juicing is loaded with powerful of vitamins, minerals and antioxidants that will do your liver great good. However, ensure your juice is made of 80- 100 percent vegetables, and the rest made of fruit.

Drink Coffee

Incredibly, coffee has many health benefits. One of which is to reduce cirrhosis (liver scarring) death by 66%. People at risk of liver disease can utilize the caffeine in coffee to lower their amount of abnormal liver enzymes. It has also been proven than people who take 3 cups of coffee a day are 25% more prone to have lower amount of liver enzymes than people who do not.

Regular Exercises

One of the ways to deal with a fatty liver is to engage in regular physical exercises. Regular exercise improves insulin resistance, helps to burn triglycerides for fuel and fights fatty liver. It is also effective for weight loss and enables you attain your desired weight. With regular exercises, an overweight or obese person can lose 3-5 % of body weight, a percentage which has been proven to improve liver condition.

However, if you are obese, it is advisable to check with your doctor before starting any exercise routine. If you aren't used to exercises, it is best to begin small with 30 minutes of aerobic activity like jogging and walking 3-5 days in a week. If you lead a sedentary lifestyle, look for how you can add more activity to your life. For instance, you could opt for the stairs instead of using the elevator or park further away from the store

As important as it is to lose weight, do not lose weight rapidly as it can worsen the liver function. It is advisable to have a gradual weight loss. This entails a 5% to 10% loss of body weight over a 6 to 12 months period, with a maximum loss of 2 pounds per week. Rapid weight loss may obstruct the bile duct, worsening your liver condition, and placing you at risk of liver disease and liver scarring.

Medication

Generally, the treatment for fatty liver is usually to control the risk factors that cause it. Therefore, people who have hypertension, diabetes and high blood cholesterol should ensure they take their prescription according to their physicians' instructions. In some cases, Vitamin E is also prescribed as an antioxidant medication.

Additionally, it is advisable to take a good liver tonic. A good liver tonic, such as Livatone Plus, will be able to repair damaged liver cells and help the liver to burn fat and rid the body of toxins. An omega-3 fatty acid supplement can also help to decrease liver fat by cutting down on the amount of unhealthy cholesterol in your body. Milk thistle and ginseng supplements are also a safe consideration because they improve the activity of liver enzyme and protect your liver from more damage.

Whatever you decide, make sure you talk it over with your physician for optimum safety. It is also safe to get a physical examination, including lab tests, liver biopsy and liver function tests to ascertain the level of the liver disease that you have.

Avoid...

- Do not try just any herbs for alternative therapy. Make sure you ask your health care provider for safe herbs to try. Some herbs, such as Artemisia, Comfrey, kava, green tea extract, mistletoe and valerian root are bad for your liver, especially if you have liver disease.

- Avoid over-the-counter medicines, especially pain-relievers with acetaminophen.

- Avoid fruit juice; it contains a high amount of carbohydrate and calories.

Recipes To Prevent And Averse Fatty Liver

BREAKFAST RECIPES

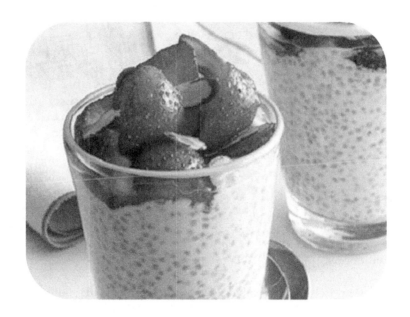

Chia-Yogurt Custard

An awesome way to start the day.

Preparation time: 10 minutes

Cooking time: 0 minute

Servings: 2

Ingredients:

1 cup of plain yogurt or kefir

¼ cup of freshly squeezed orange juice

¾ cup of coconut milk

6 tablespoons of chia seeds

2 tablespoons of honey

½ tsp ground sumac

½ tsp vanilla extract

½ tsp cinnamon

Directions:

1. Pulse the chia seeds, sumac and cinnamon in a blender until it forms a rough powder.

2. Put in the honey, yogurt, vanilla, orange juice and coconut milk. Pulse the mixture for about 4-5 times until it is thick.

3. Keep in the refrigerator, so that it can set into a custard, for an hour or overnight.

Spicy Mexican Sweet Potato Hash

A lot of veggies add a boost to your day.

Preparation time: 5 minutes

Cooking time: 10 minutes

Servings: 4

Ingredients:

1½ cups of sweet potato, skinned and chopped

1 cup of yellow corn kernels

2 tablespoons of olive oil

2 tablespoons of water

1 tablespoon of Mexican oregano

½ tablespoon of chili powder

3 garlic cloves, crushed

2 medium-sized carrots, chopped

1 large-sized jalapeno, chopped

½ medium-sized red onion

½ teaspoon of cayenne

½ teaspoon of cumin

½ teaspoon of cracked pepper

Toppings:

A squeeze of fresh lime juice

Fresh cilantro leaves

Cojita cheese, crumbled

Directions:

1. Microwave the potato with water until it's softened a bit, for 2½ minutes on high heat.

2. In a large bowl, mix the microwaved potato with jalapeno, onion, garlic, corn and carrots. Toss everything with olive oil.

3. Sprinkle the seasonings on top and stir to combine.

4. Heat a large pan over medium-high.

5. Cook the potato mixture for about 5-6 minutes or until the vegetables are slightly charred. Stir every minute.

6. Transfer to a plate; add the toppings, if desired and serve.

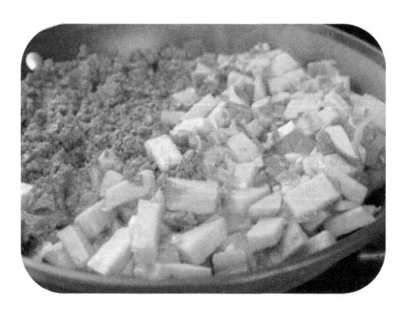

Breakfast Almond Pancakes

A highly satisfying meal.

Preparation time: 5 minutes

Cooking time: 10 minutes

Servings: 2

Ingredients:

1½ cups of almond flour

¼ cup of coconut or almond milk

2 tablespoons of coconut oil, melted

3 large eggs, whisked lightly

1 teaspoon of vanilla extract

½ teaspoon of baking soda

Few drops liquid stevia, optional

Directions:

1. Blend all the ingredients in a blender for a minute or until they are mixed thoroughly.

2. On a griddle, melt coconut oil over medium heat.

3. Heap a tablespoon with the batter and place on the griddle. Do this until all the batter is finished.

4. Cook the batter for some minutes before flipping it over.

Chinese Veggie Omelet

You can use your favorite vegetables for this omelet to suit your taste.

Preparation time: 3 minutes

Cooking time: 5 minutes

Servings: 1

Ingredients:

¼ cup of chopped kale

¼ cup of chopped green onion

¼ cup of chopped tomato

1 tablespoon of low fat sour cream

2 eggs

1 teaspoon of garlic, crushed

¼ cup of chopped mushroom, optional

¼ cup of chopped bell pepper, optional

1/8 cup of chopped serrano pepper, optional

Directions:

1. In a bowl, whisk the eggs and sour cream together until it becomes light and fluffy.

2. Sauté the kale, green onion, tomato, kale, mushroom, and peppers lightly in a small nonstick pan over medium heat for about 2-3 minutes just until it becomes soft.

3. Add in the egg mixture and cook for about 3 minutes or until you can use a spatula to lift the omelet sides from the pan.

4. Flip the omelet gently and cook for an additional 1 minute.

5. Fold the omelet in half gently and cook for 30 seconds per side.

No Grain Muesli

Super easy to prepare.

Preparation time: 5 minutes

Cooking time: 0 minute

Servings: 1

Ingredients:

½ cup of your preferred milk

2 tablespoons of unsweetened coconut, shredded

2 tablespoons of pecans, chopped

2 tablespoons of flaked almonds

1 tablespoon of chia seeds

1 tablespoon of hemp seeds

1 red apple, unpeeled, roughly grated

Pinch of clove powder

Pinch of cinnamon

Directions:

1. Thoroughly combine all the ingredients together and transfer to an airtight container. Store overnight in the refrigerator.

2. Top with fruit in the morning and eat.

Sweet Potato And Scrambled Eggs

A delightful low calorie meal.

Preparation time: 5 minutes

Cooking time: 6 minutes

Servings: 4

Ingredients:

¼ cup of canned full-fat coconut milk

8 eggs

1 large-sized cooked sweet potato, cubed

2 tablespoons of fresh parsley, minced finely

2 tablespoons of ghee or olive oil

1 teaspoon of ground cumin

1 teaspoon of dried oregano

Pepper

Salt

Directions:

1. In a large skillet, heat the ghee over medium heat.

2. In a large bowl, whisk all the ingredients except the potato. Pour this mixture into the skillet and cook until the eggs are almost done. Stir gently.

3. Add the potato cubes, stir to combine and remove from the heat.

Pecan-Ginger Cereal

Soothe your hunger and cravings with this awesome breakfast.

Preparation time: 5 minutes

Cooking time: 0 minute

Servings: 6

Ingredients:

1 cup of unsweetened coconut flakes

1 cup of toasted pecan halves

1/3 cup of toasted unsalted sunflower seeds

2 tablespoons of hemp seeds

4 dried dates, finely chopped

¼ teaspoon of dried cinnamon

¼ teaspoon of dried ginger

Directions:

1. Thoroughly combine all the ingredients and place in a glass jar.

2. Serve with milk.

Blueberry Almond Oatmeal

Delicious and filling.

Preparation time: 5 minutes

Cooking time: 30 minutes

Servings: 1

Ingredients:

1 cup of water

¼ cup of no-fat milk

¼ cup of steel-cut oats

1/3 cup of frozen or fresh blueberries

1 tablespoon of almonds

1 teaspoon of ground flaxseed

Directions:

1. Boil the water over high heat.

2. Add the oats to the boiling water and cook for 25 minutes until the oatmeal becomes soft, while stirring regularly.

3. Turn down the heat to low and cook, stirring for an extra 3 minutes.

4. Add in the remaining ingredients, combine together and serve.

Almond Bread

A heart and liver-friendly loaf.

Preparation time: 15 minutes

Cooking time: 50 minutes

Servings: 16

Ingredients:

2½ cups of almond flour

1 cup of yogurt

1 tablespoon of flax or chia seeds, ground

1 tablespoon of honey

3 eggs, separated

1 teaspoon of baking soda

¼ teaspoon of sea salt

Directions:

1. Preheat oven to 300°F.

2. Grease and flour a loaf pan with almond flour.

3. In a small bowl, mix together the flour, flaxseeds, baking soda and salt. Keep aside.

4. In another small bowl, beat the yogurt, egg yolks and honey together until it is fluffy and light. Add in the flour mixture and combine.

5. In a small bowl, let the egg whites form stiff peaks by whisking well. Fold the mixture into the dough and place in the pan.

6. Bake for 45-50 minutes or until a toothpick inserted in its middle comes out clean.

Tex-Mex SAndwich

A great breakfast that can be eaten on the go.

Preparation time: 5 minutes

Cooking time: 4 minutes

Servings: 1

Ingredients:

2 tablespoons of low-fat sharp cheddar cheese, shredded

2 slices of avocado

2 large egg whites

1 toasted multi-grain English muffin

4 teaspoons of jarred chunky salsa

Directions:

1. Grease a small non-stick pan with cooking spray and heat over medium-high.

2. Add and stir in the cheddar cheese and egg substitute.

3. Cook for 2 minutes on each side.

4. Set the eggs on the bottom half of the muffin.

5. Top with the salsa and avocado. Cover with the muffin top.

Apple Oatmeal

Combine your oat with apples and say goodbye to the doctors.

Preparation time: 5 minutes

Cooking time: 20 minutes

Servings: 1

Ingredients:

½ cup of old-fashioned rolled oats

1 medium-sized cooking apple, core removed and diced

2 tablespoons of raisins

½ tsp cinnamon

A pinch of salt

Directions:

1. Preheat oven to 350°F.

2. In a small baking dish, thoroughly mix all the ingredients together.

3. Bake for 15-20 minutes, uncovered, or until the apples are fork-tender and the mixture thickens. Stir once or twice while it bakes.

Frittata With Scallions And Salmon

Keep hunger at bay with this fiber-packed meal.

Preparation time: 7 minutes

Cooking time: 12 minutes

Servings: 6

Ingredients:

2 ounces of smoked salmon, sliced thinly and cut into ½-inch pieces

¼ cup of cold water

6 egg whites

6 scallions, trimmed and roughly chopped

4 whole eggs

2 teaspoons of extra-virgin olive oil

½ teaspoon of dried tarragon, crushed

½ cup of diced fresh basil, spinach or arugula, garnish

Directions:

1. Preheat oven to 350°F.

2. Over medium heat, heat a heavy 8-inches sauté pan for a minute. Grease the base of the pan with cooking spray; put in the olive oil and heat for 20 seconds.

3. Sauté the scallions for about 30 seconds until it becomes soft. Use a spatula to stir periodically.

4. In a medium bowl, beat the eggs, tarragon, egg whites, pepper and salt. Add this mixture to the pan.

5. Place the pieces of salmon on top and cook for about 2 minutes while stirring periodically.

6. Transfer the pan to oven and cook for about 6-8 minutes or until it turns golden, firm and puffed.

7. Using a spatula to remove from the pan, transfer the frittata onto a warm serving dish gently. Garnish with the fresh spinach if needed.

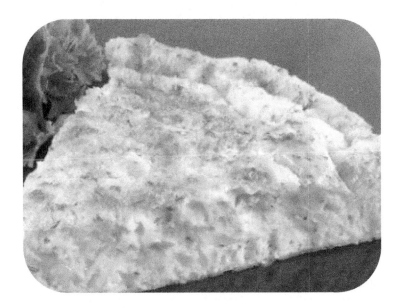

Coconut Granola

You can also have this as a snack or dessert, if you desire.

Preparation time: 5 minutes

Cooking time: 21 minutes

Servings: 4-6

Ingredients:

2 cups of no-sugar coconut chips

½ cup of almonds, chopped

½ cup of pecans, chopped

¼ cup of honey

¼ cup coconut oil

¼ cup sunflower seeds

2 tablespoons of chia seeds

1 teaspoon of ground cinnamon

½ teaspoon of ground cloves

Directions:

1. Preheat oven to 350°F.

2. In a small pot on the stove, melt the coconut oil and honey over medium heat.

3. In a large bowl, combine the remaining ingredients. Pour the coconut oil mixture over this and thoroughly mix.

4. Spread the mixture over an oven tray that has been greased or lined.

5. Bake for 15-20 minutes or until it browns lightly.

Coconut Porridge

If you are not a fan of grains, this is for you.

Preparation time: 5 minutes

Cooking time: 10 minutes

Servings: 2

Ingredients:

4 tablespoons of coconut cream

1 tablespoon of almond meal

1 tablespoon of coconut flour

1 egg, whisked lightly

Liquid stevia

Directions:

1. Put all the ingredients in a pan.

2. Cook the mixture very slowly on low while constantly stirring.

3. Serve the porridge with coconut milk

LUNCH RECIPES

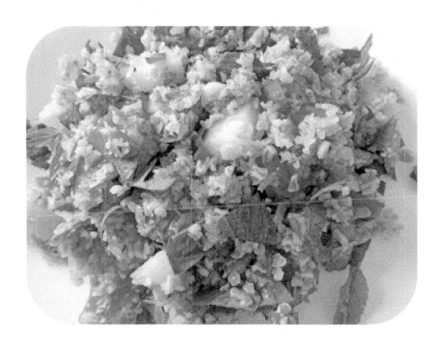

Tasty Bulgur Tabbouleh

Made with fresh veggies and packed with essential nutrients.

Preparation time: 15 minutes

Cooking time: 10 minutes

Servings: 2

Ingredients:

1 cup of vegetable stock

½ cup of chopped fresh mint

1½ cup of chopped fresh cilantro

2/3 cup of medium-fine bulgur

2 limes, juiced and zest grated

1 serrano pepper, seed removed and chopped

1 large tomato, seed removed and chopped

1 bell pepper, seed removed and chopped

1 teaspoon of olive oil

1 teaspoon of fresh ginger, grated

1 teaspoon of ancho chili powder

Directions:

1. Boil the vegetable stock in a pot.

2. Put the bulgur in a covered pan and pour the hot vegetable stock over the bulgur.

3. Cover and leave for about 15 minutes to allow the bulgur absorb the stock. Drain the excess broth and fluff the mix with a fork.

4. In the meantime, toss the spices, vegetables and herbs with the lime juice and olive oil. Allow to marinate for 5 minutes.

5. Serve with the bulgur.

Egg And Salmon Salad

A very great and quick-to-prepare recipe.

Preparation time: 15 minutes

Cooking time: 0 minute

Servings: 2

Ingredients:

6 slices of smoked salmon, sliced

4 boiled eggs, sliced

1 large handful of green beans, steamed lightly

1 large handful of arugula leaves, torn

1 Lebanese cucumber, sliced

1 small avocado, sliced

2 tablespoons of olive oil

2 tablespoons of lemon juice

Directions:

1. Put all the ingredients in a salad bowl and gently toss.

Artichoke And Chickpea Sauté

An extremely fragrant and aromatic dish.

Preparation time: 5 minutes

Cooking time: 7 minutes

Servings: 4

Ingredients:

1½ cup of artichoke hearts

1½ cup of chickpeas, cooked

2 teaspoons of turmeric

1 teaspoon of garlic, crushed

3 tablespoons of extra virgin olive oil

½ teaspoon of cracked black pepper

½ teaspoon of sea salt

Optional add-ins:

1 teaspoon of shaved ginger

1 teaspoon of coriander

1 teaspoon of fenugreek seeds

Directions:

1. Heat a large cast-iron skillet or sauté pan over medium-high.

2. In a bowl combine all the ingredients together to ensure an even coating.

3. Put the mixture in the hot skillet and shake the skillet to prevent it from sticking.

4. Cook the mixture for 5-6 minutes or until the chickpeas acquire a brown crust. Stir once a minute.

5. Squeeze lemon juice over the dish and serve.

Orange And Chicken Salad

Add a colorful and tasty flair to lunch break.

Preparation time: 10 minutes

Cooking time: 0 minute

Servings: 4

Ingredients:

¼ cup of lemon juice, freshly squeezed

4 handfuls of lettuce

2 tablespoons of olive oil

2 large ripe tomatoes, diced

2 oranges, peeled and sliced

2 celery stalks, sliced

1 Lebanese cucumber, diced

Meat from 1 cooked chicken

¼ cup of black olives, optional

Directions:

1. In a large bowl, put all the ingredients except the oil and lemon juice.

2. Drizzle the oil and lemon juice over it and toss to combine.

Cucumber Salad

Excellent for the liver and also aids digestion.

Preparation time: 12 minutes

Cooking time: 0 minute

Servings: 2

Ingredients:

For the salad:

½ cup of cherry tomatoes, cut into halves

2 Lebanese cucumbers, sliced thinly

1 large carrot, coarsely grated

2 tablespoons of fresh dill leaves, finely chopped

¼ red onion, sliced thinly

For the dressing:

2 tablespoons of olive oil

2 tablespoons of apple cider vinegar

Directions:

1. Combine all the salad ingredients in a bowl.

2. Drizzle the salad with the vinegar and olive oil

3. Toss to combine and serve.

Sweet Potato Curry

Serve this creamy dish with bread or over quinoa or rice.

Preparation time: 10 minutes

Cooking time: 25 minutes

Servings: 4

Ingredients:

1 cup of vegetable stock

1 cup of canned chickpeas

1 14-ounce can of full-fat coconut milk

3 tablespoons of curry paste

1 tablespoon of olive oil

2 handfuls of chopped fresh spinach

2 medium-size orange sweet potatoes, peeled and chopped

1 small-size brown onion, diced

1 red pepper, sliced

Directions:

1. In a large pot, heat olive oil over a stove.

2. Sauté the onion for some minutes until it is soft. Add the potato and stir thoroughly.

3. Add the curry paste and thoroughly stir. Cook for 3 minutes.

4. Put in the rest of the ingredients and leave the mixture to simmer for 20 minutes, over low heat, or until the potato is soft.

5. Serve with quinoa or rice.

Leek And Mushroom Soup

For those times when you do not feel like having a heavy lunch.

Preparation time: 25 minutes

Cooking time: 20 minutes

Servings: 4

Ingredients:

4 cups of chicken or vegetable stock

12 medium-size Swiss brown mushrooms, sliced

2 tablespoons of olive oil or ghee

3 bay leaves

2 garlic cloves, minced

½ ounce of dried porcini mushrooms

2 medium-size potatoes, peeled and diced

1 tablespoon of dried thyme leaves

2 large-size carrots, chopped

1 leek, sliced, tough ends discarded

Pepper

Salt

Directions:

1. Put the dried mushrooms in a bowl and cover with boiling water. Leave to soak for 20 minutes.

2. Heat the olive oil over medium heat in a large pot. Add the garlic and leek, sauté until tender.

3. Add in the carrots, potatoes and thyme to the pot. Cook and stir for 2 minutes.

4. Add the rest of the ingredients and allow the soup boil.

5. Turn down the heat to low and leave the soup to simmer until the veggies are soft.

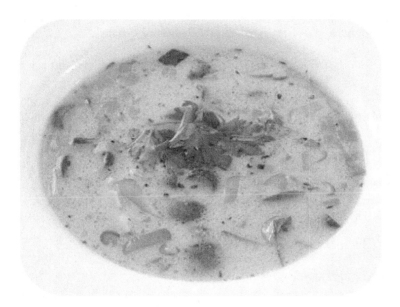

Stir Fried Lemon Chicken

This dish has an explosion of flavors that tastes just right.

Preparation time: 15 minutes

Cooking time: 18 minutes

Servings: 4

Ingredients:

10 ounces of mushrooms, cut into halves or quarters

1 pound of chicken breasts, trimmed, boneless, skinless, and cut into 1-inch pieces

1 bunch of scallions, white and green parts divided, cut into 1-inch pieces

2 cups of snow peas, stemmed and strings removed

1 cup of carrots, sliced diagonally, ¼-inch thick

½ cup of low-sodium chicken broth

3 tablespoons of low-sodium soy sauce

1 tablespoon of canola oil

1 tablespoon of garlic, chopped

2 teaspoons of cornstarch

Directions:

1. Grate a teaspoon of lemon zest and keep aside. Juice the lemon.

2. In a small bowl, whisk 3 tablespoons of the lemon juice with cornstarch, soy sauce, and broth.

3. In a large pan, heat the canola oil over medium high. Add the chicken and cook for 4-5 minutes until it is just cooked through. Stir occasionally. Use tongs to transfer to a plate.

4. Sauté the carrots and mushrooms in the pan for about 5 minutes until the carrots are just tender.

5. Add the garlic, snow peas, lemon zest and scallion whites. Cook and stir for 30 seconds until it is fragrant.

6. Whisk the lemon juice mixture, add to the skillet. Cook and stir for 2-3 minutes until it becomes thick.

7. Add the chicken with its juices and the vegetables. Cook and stir for 1-2 minutes until it is heated through.

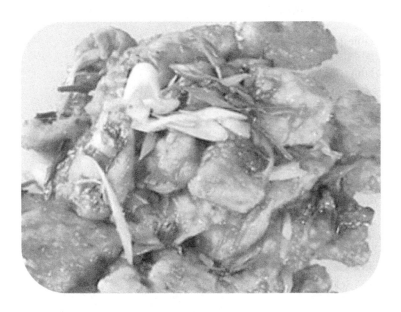

Paprika Chicken Bake

Enjoy lunch time with this baked delight.

Preparation time: 5 minutes

Cooking time: 40 minutes

Servings: 4

Ingredients:

2 pounds of pumpkin, peeled and diced

2 pounds of chicken thighs and drumsticks pieces

¼ cup of pine nuts

4 tablespoons of olive oil

1 tablespoon of paprika powder

1 rosemary sprig

Pepper

Salt

Directions:

1. Preheat oven to 400°F.

2. Grease an oven dish and place the pumpkin and chicken pieces in it. Use a pastry brush to brush them with oil.

3. Sprinkle the paprika, pepper and salt over the pumpkin and chicken evenly. Add the sprig of rosemary.

4. Use a foil to cover the dish and place in the oven. Bake for 30 minutes.

5. Remove the foil, add the nuts and keep baking until the chicken is well-cooked.

DINNER RECIPES

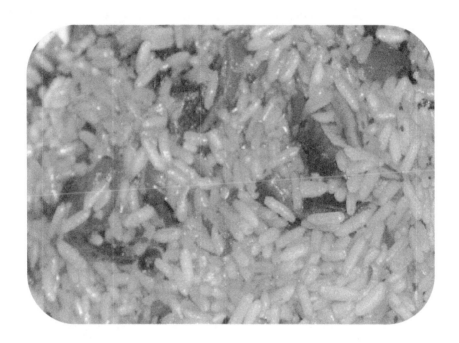

Herby Rice-Mushroom Casserole

This dish feels light but it's actually really filling.

Preparation time: 5 minutes

Cooking time: 46 minutes

Servings: 3

Ingredients:

4 cups of diced cremini, Portobello, trumpet or oyster mushroom

2 cups of cooked brown rice

1½ cups of vegetable stock

5 green onion, white and green parts only, chopped

2 medium bunches of dill, stemmed and crushed

1 medium brunch of fresh parsley, stemmed and crushed

2 tablespoons of olive oil

1 teaspoon of crushed garlic

1 teaspoon of dried oregano

½ teaspoon of cayenne pepper

½ teaspoon of ground black pepper

Directions:

1. Heat the oil in a large pan over medium heat. Sauté and stir the garlic and onions for about 5 minutes until the onions are translucent.

2. Add the oregano, cayenne and black pepper and cook an extra minute.

3. Add in the mushrooms, parsley and dill. Cook for about 5-10 minutes until the mushrooms are soft.

4. Preheat oven to 350°F.

5. Mix the vegetables with the cooked rice in a casserole dish and pour the stock over it.

6. Uncover and bake for 30 minutes.

Thai Red Snapper
The flavors in this dish are amazingly intense.

Preparation time: 10 minutes

Cooking time: 15 minutes

Servings: 4

Ingredients:

1½ pounds of red snapper

8 shallots, crushed

2 limes, cut in halves

2 tablespoons of crushed garlic

2 tablespoons of peanut oil

2 tablespoons of crushed ginger

1 dried red chili, crumbled

2 teaspoons of turmeric

½ teaspoon of sea salt flakes, divided

Directions:

1. Toss the snapper in the turmeric and keep aside.

2. Grind the shallots with half of the salt into a paste using a mortar and pestle. Transfer to a bowl.

3. Grind the remaining salt with garlic and ginger in the mortar.

4. Heat a large pan over medium heat. Cook the shallot paste with ½ tablespoon of oil for about 5 minutes until it is lightly brown.

5. Add the garlic mixture and chili. Cook for an extra 5 minutes.

6. Add the remaining peanut oil and then the fish. Cook for 1½-2 minutes.

7. Turn the pieces over and cook for an extra 1½-2 minutes.

8. Remove from heat and squeeze the lime over the meal.

Basil Chicken Stir-Fry

An excellent dinner choice.

Preparation time: 5 minutes

Cooking time: 15 minutes

Servings: 4

Ingredients:

1 pound of ground chicken

4 tablespoons of lime juice, freshly squeezed

2 tablespoons of olive oil

1 tablespoon of soy sauce, tamari or coconut aminos

1 tablespoon of fish sauce

1 large handful fresh basil leaves

1 red pepper, sliced

Directions:

1. In a large pan, heat the olive oil. Stir-fry the chicken for some minutes until it is well-cooked.

2. Add the pepper and also stir-fry for some minutes.

3. Add the remaining ingredients except the basil.

4. Throw in the basil, stir to combine and remove from heat.

Maple And Lemon Roasted Sweet Potatoes
Tasty and healthy.

Preparation time: 10 minutes

Cooking time: 1 hour 15 minutes

Servings: 16

Ingredients:

2½ lb sweet potatoes, peeled & cut into cubes of 1½-inches

1/3 cup of pure maple syrup

1 red onion, large-sized, halved across the length & cut diagonally into slices of ¼ inches, optional

2 tablespoons of olive oil

1 tablespoon of lemon juice, freshly squeezed

Directions:

1. Preheat oven to 400°F

2. In a small bowl, mix the maple syrup, lemon juice, olive oil, salt and pepper.

3. Put the onions and potatoes in a baking dish and drizzle the syrup mixture over it. Toss the mixture to coat and spread out the potatoes uniformly to cover the dish.

4. Cover with foil and bake for 15 minutes.

5. Uncover and stir. Cook for an hour or until the potatoes are soft and begin to brown. Stir every 15 minutes.

Turkey Meatloaf

A unique liver-friendly version of the classic meatloaf made with beef.

Preparation time: 15 minutes

Cooking time: 1 hour

Servings: 8

Ingredients:

2 pounds of lean ground turkey breast

1 8-ounce can of unsalted tomato sauce

½ cup of no-fat milk

½ cup of red or orange bell pepper, seed removed and finely diced

¼ cup of ketchup

¾ cup of quick cooking oats

2 large eggs, beaten

1 medium onion, finely diced

2 teaspoons of Worcestershire sauce

½ teaspoon of salt

Freshly ground black pepper

Directions:

46

1. Preheat oven to 350°F.

2. Combine the milk and oats in a small bowl. Leave for at least 3 minutes to soak.

3. Mix the oats mixture with the remaining ingredients except the tomato sauce in a large bowl.

4. Transfer into a 9 x 13 baking dish to form a loaf shape. Pour the tomato sauce over the loaf.

5. Bake for about 1 hour.

Greek-Style Lamb Meatballs

Delicious, healthy and juicy.

Preparation time: 15 minutes

Cooking time: 20 minutes

Servings: 4

Ingredients:

1½ pounds of ground lamb

¼ cup of feta cheese, diced

1 tablespoon of dried oregano

2 garlic cloves, crushed

1 handful fresh parsley, finely chopped

1 egg, whisked lightly

1 teaspoon of dried rosemary

½ teaspoon of salt

Directions:

1. Preheat oven to 350°F.

2. In a large bowl, mix all the ingredients thoroughly with your hands.

3. Shape the mixture into meat balls and arrange them on a greased or lined baking tray.

4. Bake for 20 minutes.

Ginger Spiced Chicken

Spice-up your meal with this great chicken delight.

Preparation time: 5 minutes

Cooking time: 40 minutes

Servings: 4

Ingredients:

1½ pounds of chicken drumsticks

1 tablespoon of olive oil or ghee

1 small brown onion, chopped

1 inch of sliced fresh ginger, peeled and chopped finely

½ red pepper, sliced

½ teaspoon of salt

½ teaspoon of cayenne pepper

Directions:

1. In a pan over medium heat, put the oil.

2. Sauté the onion and garlic for 3 minutes.

3. Add the rest of the ingredients except the chicken.

4. Add the chicken, combine and reduce the heat to simmer gently.

5. Cook for 30 minutes or until the chicken is well-cooked. Stir occasionally.

Browned Salmon

Wonderful and simple to prepare.

Preparation time: 10 minutes

Cooking time: 10 minutes

Servings: 4

Ingredients:

4 fillets salmon

2 tablespoons of capers

2 tablespoons of olive oil

4 lemon slices

1/8 teaspoon of ground black pepper

1/8 teaspoon of salt

Directions:

1. Preheat a large heavy pan for 3 minutes over medium heat.

2. Use oil to coat salmon and place in the pan. Turn up the heat to high and cook for 3 minutes.

3. Sprinkle the capers, pepper and salt on the salmon, flip and cook for 5 minutes or until it is browned.

4. Garnish the salmon with lemon slices.

Portobello Steak

This dish substitutes the meat with mushrooms.

Preparation time: 10 minutes

Cooking time: 18 minutes

Servings: 4

Ingredients:

3 ounces of low-fat provolone or vegan cheese, sliced thinly

4 large Portobello mushrooms, stemmed, gills removed and sliced

4 whole-wheat rolls, split and toasted

¼ cup of vegetable broth

1 tablespoon of all-purpose flour

1 tablespoon of low-sodium soy sauce

2 teaspoons of dried oregano

2 teaspoons of extra virgin olive oil

1 medium onion, sliced

1 large red pepper, sliced thinly

½ teaspoon of freshly ground pepper

Directions:

1. In a large nonstick pan, heat the olive oil over medium-high heat. Sauté the onion for about 5 minutes until it is tender and starts to brown. Stir often.

2. Add the bell pepper, mushrooms, red pepper and oregano. Cook for about 7 minutes until the veggies are tender and wilts. Stir often.

3. Turn down heat to low, sprinkle the flour on the vegetables and stir to combine. Stir in the soy sauce and broth. Bring the mixture to simmer.

4. Remove from heat and place the slices of cheese on top of the vegetables. Cover and leave to stand for 1-2 minutes until it melts.

5. Use a spatula to divide the mixture into 4 portions. Leave the melted cheese on top.

6. Spoon a portion onto each bun and serve.

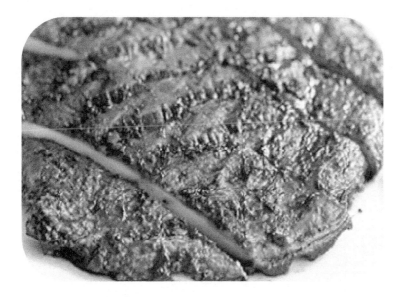

SNACKS

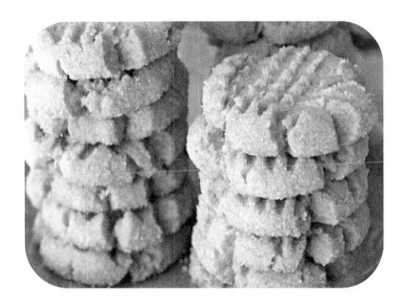

Coconut Cashew Honey Cookies

Appease your sweet buds with these yummy cookies.

Preparation time: 15 minutes

Cooking time: 25 minutes

Servings: 12

Ingredients:

1 cup of rolled oats

1 cup of unsweetened coconut, shredded

½ cup of coconut oil

½ cup of local honey

½ cup of cashews, finely ground

½ cup of almond flour

¼ cup of almond or coconut milk

¼ cup of whole wheat flour

1 tablespoon of lecithin

½ teaspoon of salt

Directions:

1. Preheat oven to 350°F.

2. Cream the coconut oil, honey, ground cashew, almond flour, lecithin together.

3. Add the oats, shredded coconut, whole wheat flour and salt. Combine thoroughly.

4. Pour in the milk and stir until it is smooth.

5. Line a baking sheet with parchment paper and drop the dough on it with two spoons.

6. Bake for 20-25 minutes.

Italian Quinoa Bites

Everybody sure loves this Italian treat.

Preparation time: 7 minutes

Cooking time: 20 minutes

Servings: 12

Ingredients:

1 cup of cooked quinoa

½ cup of zucchini, shredded

½ cup of grated Asiago cheese

½ cup of sun-dried tomatoes, finely diced

2 large eggs

1 egg white

2 tablespoons of diced green onions

2 tablespoons of diced parsley

1 tablespoon of diced basil

Cracked black pepper

Sea salt

Directions:

1. Preheat oven to 350°F.

2. Thoroughly mix all the ingredients in a large bowl.

3. Grease a mini-muffin pan lightly and spoon the mixture into the pan evenly.

4. Bake for 15-20 minutes until the muffins turn golden brown.

Banana Muffins

Dairy-free, oil-free and sugar-free.

Preparation time: 5 minutes

Cooking time: 20 minutes

Servings: 8-9

Ingredients:

1 can of white beans, rinsed thoroughly and patted dry

½ cup of quinoa flakes or quick oats, loosely packed

¼ cup of honey or maple syrup

¼ cup of peanut butter

1 medium overripe banana, mashed

2 teaspoons of pure vanilla extract

¼ teaspoon of salt

¾ teaspoon of baking powder

1/8 teaspoon of baking soda

Directions:

1. Preheat oven to 350°F. Line about 8 to 9 muffin cups.

2. Process all the ingredients in a food processor or blender until it is smooth.

3. Pour the mixture into the muffin cups. Be careful not to overfill the cups.

4. Bake for 20 minutes

Oat Cookies

A tasty treat made with just five ingredients.

Preparation time: 10 minutes

Cooking time: 10 minutes

Servings: 12

Ingredients:

2 cups of rolled oats

1/3 cup of no-sugar coconut flakes

¼ cup of sunflower seeds

¼ cup of pumpkin seeds

3 large over-ripe bananas, mashed

Directions:

1. Preheat oven to 350°F.

2. Blend the oats in a food processor until they resemble flour.

3. Mix the oat flour with the remaining ingredients and leave to stand for 2 minutes.

4. Bake for 10 minutes until they turn lightly golden and are set.

Potato Chips

Microwave made chips with an unforgettable great taste.

Preparation time: 10 minutes

Cooking time: 7 minutes

Servings: 4

Ingredients:

1 1/3 pounds of red or Yukon Gold potatoes, unpeeled, scrubbed and cut into thin 1/8-inch slices.

½ teaspoon of salt

2 teaspoons of extra virgin olive oil

Directions:

1. In a medium bowl, evenly toss the potato slices with the olive oil and salt to coat.

2. With cooking spray, grease a large microwave-proof plate.

3. Arrange the slices of potato on the plate in a single layer.

4. Microwave for 2-3 minutes on high while uncovered. Flip the slices and keep microwaving for 2-4 minutes until the edges begin to brown and turn crispy.

Apricot Canapés

Impossible to stop at one bite.

Preparation time: 10 minutes

Cooking time: 0 minute

Servings: 16

Ingredients:

2 ounces of pistachios, chopped and shelled

8 teaspoons of blue cheese, crumbled

½ teaspoon of honey

16 dried apricots

Freshly ground pepper

Directions:

1. Top each of the apricots with ½ teaspoon of cheese.

2. Sprinkle the apricots with pistachios.

3. Drizzle honey over it and sprinkle with pepper.

Apple Crumble

Satisfy your mid-day cravings with this yummy snack.

Preparation time: 5 minutes

Cooking time: 30 minutes

Servings: 6

Ingredients:

2 cups of cooked quinoa

4 large apples, peeled, core removed and chopped

1 cup of flour

½ cup of chopped pecans, cashews or walnuts

1/3 cup of ground almonds

2 teaspoons of cinnamon

Directions:

1. Preheat oven to 350°F.

2. Oil a baking dish lightly and place the apples in them.

3. In a medium bowl, combine the remaining ingredients. Crumble this mixture over the apples top.

4. Bake for 30 minutes or until the crumble is browned lightly and the apples are soft.

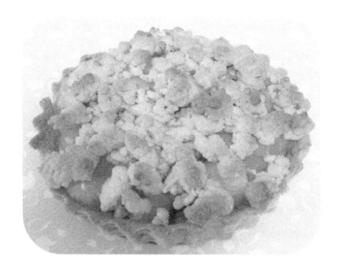

Roasted Cumin Carrots

Maximize all the benefits from carrots with this crunchy snack.

Preparation time: 10 minutes

Cooking time: 30 minutes

Servings: 4

Ingredients:

1 pound of carrots, peeled

1½ tablespoons of ghee

½ tablespoon of ground cumin

¼ teaspoon of salt

½ teaspoon of dried oregano

Directions:

1. Preheat oven to 400°F.

2. Divide the carrots in halves and cut in halves again lengthwise.

3. Arrange the carrot pieces on a greased or lined baking tray.

4. In a small bowl, combine the butter with cumin, salt and oregano. Brush this mixture over the carrots until they are well coated.

5. Roast the carrots for 15-30 minutes or until it is tender and browned lightly.

Peach Crumble

No artificial sweeteners.

Preparation time: 10 minutes

Cooking time: 45 minutes

Servings: 9

Ingredients:

4 extra-large peaches, chopped

¼ cup of whole wheat flour

¾ cup of old-fashioned oats

2 tablespoons of coconut oil

2 tablespoons of agave

2 tablespoons of cornstarch

1½ teaspoon of almond extract, alcohol-free

1 teaspoon of ground cinnamon, divided

Directions:

1. Preheat oven to 350°F.

2. Thoroughly mix the peaches, almond extract, cornstarch and ¼ teaspoon of cinnamon in a medium bowl.

3. In another bowl, combine the remaining cinnamon with flour and oats.

4. Add the coconut oil and agave. Combine until it is thoroughly mixed.

5. Spread the peach mixture into a baking dish and sprinkle the oats mixture evenly on top.

6. Bake for 35-45 minutes or until the oat mixture becomes crunchy and the peach juice is bubbling.

SOUPS

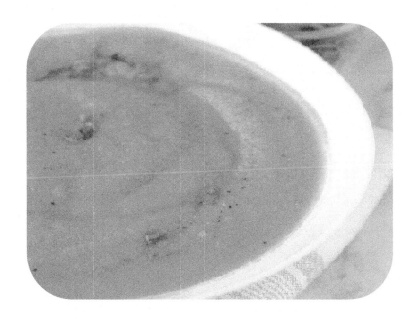

Ginger And Carrot Soup

A bowl of comfort.

Preparation time: 6 minutes

Cooking time: 10 minutes

Servings: 4

Ingredients:

5 cups of vegetable stock or water

2 tablespoons of canned full-fat coconut milk

1 tablespoon of olive oil

8 carrots, peeled and chopped

2 parsnips, peeled and chopped

2 zucchinis, chopped

1 inch of fresh ginger, peeled and grated

1 teaspoon of ground turmeric

Pepper

Salt

Directions:

1. In a large pot, heat oil over medium heat. Gently sauté the parsnips and carrots for 3 minutes.

2. Add the remaining ingredients and simmer over low heat until the veggies are soft.

Mushroom Soup

You will never go for can soup after this.

Preparation time: 10 minutes

Cooking time: 37 minutes

Servings: 4

Ingredients:

20 stalks of fresh thyme, leaves removed

2 10-ounce packages of baby Portobello mushroom, sliced

2 10-ounce packages of white button mushroom, sliced

2 cups of unsweetened cashew or almond milk

2 cups of organic vegetable broth

2 tablespoons of tapioca flour

1 tablespoon of soy sauce or liquid aminos

2 large white onions, chopped

2 dried bay leaves

1 teaspoon of salt

Freshly ground black pepper

Directions:

1. Add the onions to a large saucepan, cover and sweat them for 5-7 minutes over medium heat.

2. Shift the onion to the pan sides and add the mushrooms to the center. Uncover and cook for 5 minutes.

3. Combine the mushrooms and onions together.

4. Add the thyme and keep cooking for at least 10 minutes.

5. Add the tapioca into the broth in a small bowl and stir until it is mixed and does not have lumps. Pour this mix into the mushrooms and stir to combine.

6. Add the milk to the pan and cook for at least 15 minutes while stirring occasionally.

7. Taste and season with salt and pepper.

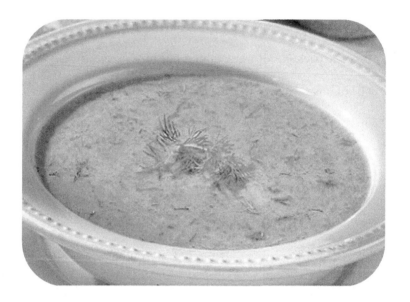

Detox Broccoli Soup

Green, delicious and comforting.

Preparation time: 10 minutes

Cooking time: 15 minutes

Servings: 6

Ingredients:

2 cups of low sodium vegetable broth or filtered water

2 cups of broccoli florets

1 cup of greens

1 tablespoon of chia seeds

2 celery stalks, chopped finely

2 cloves of garlic, minced

1 carrot, peeled and chopped finely

1 onion, finely chopped

1 parsnip, peeled and chopped finely

Juice of ½ a lemon

1 teaspoon of coconut oil

½ teaspoon of sea salt

1 teaspoon of coconut milk, garnish

Mixed nuts and seeds, toasted

Directions:

1. Heat the oil in a soup pot over low heat and sauté the onion, parsnip, garlic, broccoli, carrot, and celery sticks for 5 minutes. Stir frequently.

2. Add the broth and allow to boil. Cover the pot and leave to simmer for 5-7 minutes until the vegetables are soft but not mushy.

3. Add the greens and stir. Transfer the soup to a blender, add the lemon and chia seeds and blend into a smooth cream.

4. Top the soup with the nuts and seeds.

Healthy Vegetable Soup
A nutritious soup loaded with minerals, vitamins and fiber.

Preparation time: 15 minutes

Cooking time: 20 minutes

Servings: 8

Ingredients:

4 cups of vegetable broth

4 plum Roma tomatoes, peeled, seeded and chopped

3 garlic cloves, minced or chopped

1 yellow onion, diced

1 zucchini, halved lengthwise and sliced thinly crosswise

1 carrot, peeled, halved lengthwise and sliced thinly crosswise

1 bay leaf

1 yellow bell pepper, seeded and chopped

2 tablespoons of diced fresh cilantro

1 tablespoon of olive oil

1 tablespoon of diced fresh oregano

1 tablespoon of lemon zest, grated

1 teaspoon of ground cumin

¼ teaspoon of freshly ground pepper

¼ teaspoon of salt

Directions:

1. Heat the oil in a large saucepan over medium heat. Sauté the onions for about 4 minutes until they are tender and translucent.

2. Sauté the garlic for 30 seconds, ensure that it does not brown. Sauté the oregano, tomatoes and cumin for about 4 minutes until the tomatoes are soft.

3. Add the bay leaf and broth and allow to boil. Turn down the heat to medium-low and leave to simmer.

4. Add and cook the bell pepper and carrot for 2 minutes.

5. Add the zucchini and simmer for about 3 minutes until the vegetables are soft.

6. Add the cilantro and lemon zest, and stir.

7. Add salt and pepper to season.

8. Remove bay leaf and serve.

Beet Soup

A healthy soup for the liver.

Preparation time: 15 minutes

Cooking time: 37 minutes

Servings: 2

Ingredients:

2 cups of warm vegetable broth

3 medium beet roots

2 cloves of garlic, minced

2 carrots, finely chopped

1 small leek, finely chopped

1 tablespoon of sunflower, chia and pumpkin seeds

1 teaspoon of coconut oil

¼ teaspoon of sea salt

1 teaspoon of coconut milk, garnish

Directions:

1. Put the beets in a pot, cover it with water and allow to boil then simmer for 30 minutes until it is soft. Drain and keep aside

2. In a skillet, heat the coconut oil over low heat and sauté the leek, garlic, carrot and onions for 5-7 minutes. Remove from heat and put in a plate.

3. Peel the beets and cut into cubes. Put in a blender alongside the broth and cooked vegetables. Blend into a smooth cream.

4. Season with salt.

5. Garnish with the seeds and serve.

Lentil And Kale Soup

Contains the superfood– kale.

Preparation time: 5 minutes

Cooking time: 20 minutes

Servings: 4-6

Ingredients:

1 bunch of kale, stemmed and coarsely chopped

8 cups of vegetable stock

1½ cups of red lentils, rinsed

1 tablespoon of chopped parsley

2 onions, chopped

2 carrots, chopped

1 garlic clove

Zest of ½ a lemon

¼ teaspoon of red pepper flakes, optional

Directions:

1. Put the kale, lentils, stock, garlic, onions and carrots in a large pot. Allow to boil and cook for about 15-20 minutes until the lentils are soft.

2. Add the pepper flakes, lemon zest and parsley. Stir and serve.

Vegetarian Detox Soup

The perfect choice for detoxing.

Preparation time: 15 minutes

Cooking time: 35 minutes

Servings: 8

Ingredients:

4 cups of filtered or spring water

1 pound of fresh green beans

4 medium zucchini

3-4 green onions, spring onions, scallions

3 celery stalks

3 garlic cloves

3 tomatoes

4-6 kale leaves

2 carrots

1 handful of coriander, cilantro, Chinese parsley

1 bunch of fresh Italian flat-leaf parsley

1 avocado, sliced

3 tablespoons of tamari or liquid aminos

2 tablespoons of seaweed flakes

2 tablespoons of amaranth or teff seeds, optional

Directions:

1. Wash all the vegetables and pulse each of them in the food processor until they are all chopped finely.

2. Add the vegetables to a large, heavy bottom pot as you chop.

3. Pour in the water and add the tamari, seaweed or amaranth seeds, if desired.

4. Allow to boil, reduce the heat, cover the pot and leave to gently simmer for 30 minutes.

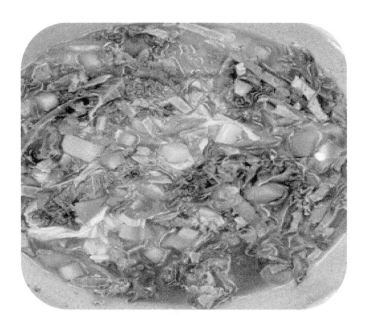

Chicken Soup

A fantastic soup that is great for the liver.

Preparation time: 15 minutes

Cooking time: 35 minutes

Servings: 8-12 minutes

Ingredients:

2 quarts of chicken broth

3 cups of broccoli florets

2 cups of celery, diced

2½ cups of carrots, sliced

1½ cups of frozen peas

¼ cup of parsley, diced

1½ pounds of chicken breast, boneless and skinless

3 tablespoons of fresh ginger, shredded or grated

3-4 garlic cloves, crushed

2 tablespoons of olive oil

1 tablespoon of apple cider vinegar

1 large onion, peeled and diced

¼ teaspoon of ground turmeric

¼ - ½ teaspoon of crushed red pepper

Pepper

Salt

Directions:

1. Place a large pot over medium heat and add the oil, ginger, onions, garlic and celery. Sauté the veggies for 5-6 minutes until they tender.

2. Add the broth, chicken, vinegar, red pepper, carrots, turmeric and a teaspoon of salt. Boil, reduce the heat and simmer for 20 minutes until the chicken are well-cooked. Use tongs to remove the chicken onto a cutting board and allow to cool.

3. Add the peas, broccoli and parsley to the pot and keep on simmering until the broccoli is soft.

4. In the meantime, shred the chicken with two forks, add it back to the pot and stir.

5. Adjust seasoning when the broccoli is soft.

SALADS

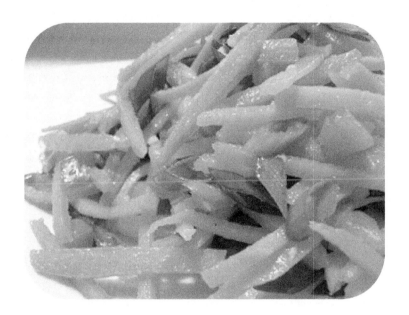

Detox Salad

Put your liver back on track with this salad.

Preparation time: 20 minutes

Cooking time: 0 minute

Servings: 4

Ingredients:

For the dressing:

4 tablespoons of light olive oil

2 tablespoons of lemon juice, freshly squeezed

2 teaspoons of ginger root, grated

1 teaspoon of honey

For the salad:

3 carrots, roughly grated

2 Gala apples, cut into quarters, cored and sliced

2 celery sticks or a handful of radishes, sliced

½ medium head of shredded red cabbage

3 tablespoons of pine nuts, toasted

2 tablespoons of flax seed

2 tablespoons of fresh parsley, coarsely chopped

2 tablespoons of sunflower seeds

1 tablespoon of pumpkin seeds

Directions:

1. Mix all the salad ingredients in a large bowl.

2. Whisk the dressing ingredients in a small bowl until it thickens.

3. Drizzle the dressing over the salad and toss to coat.

Ginger And Carrot Salad
Made with fresh ingredients and packed with flavors.

Preparation time: 12 minutes

Cooking time: 0 minute

Servings: 2-4

Ingredients:

For the salad:

3 medium carrots, roughly grated

2 tablespoons of sesame seeds, dry roasted lightly

1 cup of fresh bean sprouts, optional

For the dressing:

¼ cup of lemon juice, freshly squeezed

4 teaspoons of brown or palm sugar

3 teaspoons of fresh ginger, finely grated

1 dessert spoon of sesame oil

1 dessert spoon of peanut oil

Freshly ground black pepper

Directions:

1. Whisk the dressing ingredients in a bowl and drizzle over the salad ingredients. Toss to coat.

Kale-Blueberry Salad

Wipe the slate clean with this super salad combo.

Preparation time: 10 minutes

Cooking time: 0 minute

Servings: 2

Ingredients:

½ cup of cooked quinoa

½ cup of blueberries

¼ cup of slivered almonds

4 stalks of raw kale, washed and chopped into bite-size pieces

1 tablespoon of extra virgin olive oil

½ tablespoon of honey

Juice of 1 large lemon

1 teaspoon of poppy seeds

Directions:

1. Whisk the oil, honey and lemon in a small bowl. Keep aside.

2. Put the blueberries, kale, almonds and quinoa in a large bowl.

3. Drizzle the dressing on the salad and toss to coat well.

4. Add the poppy seeds and toss to combine.

Kale Salad With Apple Lemon Dressing

Harness the powers of kale in this delicious salad.

Preparation time: 10 minutes

Cooking time: 0 minute

Servings: 2-4

Ingredients:

For the Dressing:

2 tablespoons of apple cider vinegar

2 tablespoons of olive oil

1 tablespoon of lemon juice

1 teaspoon of honey

For the Salad:

½ cup of chopped red onion

½ cup of dried cranberries

¼ cup of pine nuts

1 bunch of kale, stemmed and chopped

Directions:

1. Whisk the dressing ingredients in a bowl thoroughly.

2. Add the kale to the dressing and massage for several minutes.

3. Add the remaining ingredients once the kale has absorbed the dressing. Toss everything to combine.

Green Goddess Salad

Cleanse your system with this healthy salad.

Preparation time: 10 minutes

Cooking time: 0 minute

Servings: 4

Ingredients:

Dressing:

½ cup of packed cilantro

¼ cup of olive oil

2/3 cup of Greek yogurt

1 tablespoon of agave nectar

2 scallions

1 lime, juiced

½ jalapeno pepper

½ teaspoon of salt

½ teaspoon of garlic, minced

Salad:

4 cups of spinach

1-2 cups of pea shoots

½ cups of chopped or crushed almonds

½ cup of feta cheese

1 avocado, chunked

Directions:

1. Puree all the dressing ingredients until you get the right texture. Add the cilantro last.

2. Toss the salad with the dressing and serve.

Winter Detox Salad

Mesmerizing colors and amazing taste.

Preparation time: 10 minutes

Cooking time: 0 minute

Servings: 4

Ingredients:

¼ cup of walnut pieces

¼ cup of fennel, sliced thinly or shaved

2 tangerines, peeled and segmented + 1 for dressing

1 small bunch of raw or blanched broccoli

1 avocado, sliced

1 pomegranate, seed removed

Extra virgin olive oil

Directions:

1. In a medium bowl, toss all the ingredients together except the olive oil.

2. Drizzle one juiced tangerine and olive oil over the salad.

3. Season with salt and pepper.

Salmon, Spinach And Blueberries Salad

Insanely delicious and healthy.

Preparation time: 10 minutes

Cooking time: 0 minute

Servings: 2

Ingredients:

8 ounces of smoked salmon, coarsely chopped

4 cups of mixed greens or baby spinach

½ cup of fresh blueberries

¼ cup of light blue or feta cheese, crumbled

½ red onion, sliced thinly

¼ cup of chopped walnuts, optional

1 avocado, peeled, pit removed and chopped

Directions:

1. Combine all the ingredients together and toss with vinaigrette.

Amazing Detox Salad

Get rid of all the harmful toxins in your body with this magical salad.

Preparation time: 10 minutes

Cooking time: 20 minutes

Servings: 4

Ingredients:

2 cups of loosely packed fresh baby spinach

1 cup of cherry tomatoes, cut into halves

1 cup of quinoa

3 tablespoons of olive oil

2 tablespoons of raw whole almond

2 tablespoons of raw cashews

2 tablespoons of lemon juice, freshly squeezed

1 tablespoon of white balsamic vinegar

2 large sweet potatoes, cut into ½-inch cubes

1 head of broccoli, cut into florets

1 small head of red cabbage, shredded

Sea salt

Pepper

Directions:

1. Cook the quinoa following package instructions.

2. In the meantime, steam the potatoes and broccoli in a steamer basket for 10 minutes over medium heat until soft.

3. Combine the potatoes, broccoli, cabbage, quinoa and spinach in a large bowl.

4. Whisk the lemon juice, oil and vinegar in a small bowl and drizzle over the salad.

5. Add the almonds and cashews. Toss to mix.

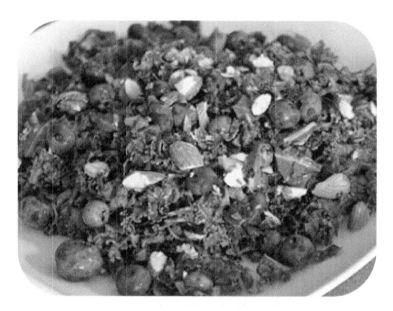

Kale blueberry Salad

DRINKS

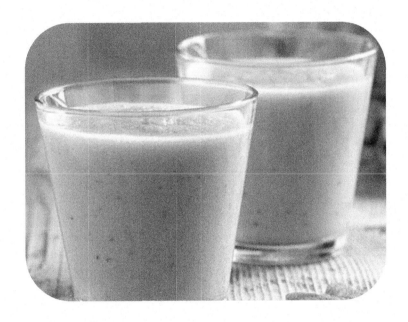

Turmeric Tea

Boost your overall immunity with this special tea.

Preparation time: 2 minutes

Cooking time: 3 minutes

Servings: 2

Ingredients:

2 cups of milk

1 teaspoon of honey

1 teaspoon of turmeric

½ tsp cinnamon

¼ teaspoon of ground ginger powder

A pinch of black pepper

Directions:

1. Process all the ingredients in a blender until it is smooth.

2. Pour the mixture into a saucepan and heat over medium heat for 3 minutes until it gets hot but not boiling. Drink while hot.

Green Detox Drink

An effective way of detoxifying the liver.

Preparation time: 5 minutes

Cooking time: 0 minute

Servings: 1

Ingredients:

2 cups of kale

1 cup of Swiss chard

1 lime peeled

½ lemon, peeled

½ cucumber

Directions:

1. Process all the ingredients in a juicer and drink.

Ginger Apple Drink

This drink promotes blood circulation.

Preparation time: 5 minutes

Cooking time: 0 minute

Servings: 1-2

Ingredients:

2 celery stalks

2 large green apples, cored

2 medium ginger pieces

2 large carrots

1 tablespoon of hemp oil

A pinch of turmeric powder

Directions:

1. Run the celery, ginger, apple and carrot through a juicer.

2. Pour mixture into glass and stir in the hemp oil and turmeric.

3. Serve drink over ice.

Veggie Fruit Smoothies
Your daily nutritional requirements all in one glass.

Preparation time: 5 minutes

Cooking time: 0 minute

Servings: 2-3

Ingredients:

2 cups of coconut water

1 cup of spinach

1 cup of watercress

4 celery stalks

2 carrots

1 garlic clove

1 red bell pepper

1 large tomato

1 red jalapeno, seeded, optional

Directions:

1. Process all the ingredients in a food processor or blender.

Watermelon Juice

This healthy drink contains all the vitamins you need.

Preparation time: 5 minutes

Cooking time: 0 minute

Servings: 1

Ingredients:

1 handful of fresh mint leaves

1 large carrot

1 cup of watermelon, cut into cubes

1 Lebanese cucumber

Directions:

1. Run all the ingredients through a juicer.

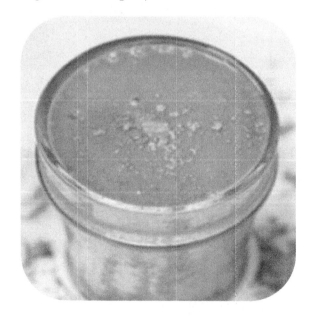

Banana-Cacao Shake

Shamrock Shake

A drink that prevents constipation and aids detoxification.

Preparation time: 3 minutes

Cooking time: 0 minute

Servings: 2

Ingredients:

1 scoop of Ultra Nourish superfood shake

2 cups of frozen vanilla yogurt

½ teaspoon of alcohol-free mint extract

1½ cups of vanilla almond milk

Directions:

1. Blend the ingredients in a blender until it is smooth.

Banana Cacao Shake

A nutrient-dense smoothie.

Preparation time: 5 minutes

Cooking time: 0 minute

Servings: 1

Ingredients:

1 cup of almond milk

3 tablespoons of whey protein powder

2 tablespoons of cocoa or cacao powder

1 tablespoon of almond butter

1 frozen banana, chopped

Cacao nibs, optional

Directions:

1. Blend all the ingredients in a blender until smooth.

2. Sprinkle with cacao nibs, if desired.

Pumpkin Spiced Latte

Forget about buying this autumn favorite and make your own.

Preparation time: 5 minutes

Cooking time: 5 minutes

Servings: 1

Ingredients:

8 ounces of coffee, freshly brewed

½ cup of unsweetened vanilla almond milk

2-3 drops of liquid stevia

3 tablespoons of pumpkin puree

1 teaspoon of pumpkin pie spice

½ teaspoon of alcohol free vanilla

A sprinkle of cinnamon

Directions:

1. Combine the pumpkin puree and milk in a saucepan or cup. Cook on stove over medium heat until it is hot but not boiling.

2. Remove from the heat, add the vanilla, cinnamon, pumpkin spice and stevia. Stir.

3. Blend the mixture for 30 seconds in a blender or until it foams.

4. Pour coffee into a mug, add the blended mixture and sprinkle cinnamon on top.

Super Detox Smoothie

A satisfying and filling smoothie.

Preparation time: 5 minutes

Cooking time: 0 minute

Servings: 2

Ingredients:

2 cups of coconut water

1 cup of mixed greens

¼ cup of parsley or coriander

1 zucchini, chopped and frozen

1 small green apple, chopped and frozen

Juice of ½ lemon

¼ avocado, chopped and frozen

1 tsp chia seeds

¼ teaspoon of ground turmeric

Directions:

1. Blend all the ingredients in a blender for 30 seconds or until it is smooth.

DESSERTS

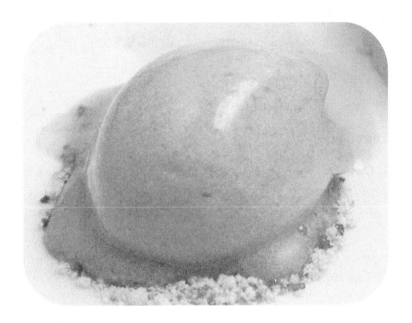

Raspberry-Pineapple Parfaits
A healthy dessert with low calories.

Preparation time: 5 minutes

Cooking time: 0 minute

Servings: 4

Ingredients:

2 cups of nonfat peach yogurt

1½ cups of pineapple chunks

1¼ cups of fresh raspberries

Directions:

1. Divide the ingredients among 4 glasses. Layer them starting with the yogurt, raspberries and pineapple.

Apple Cucumber Sorbet
Delicious, simple and healthy.

Preparation time: 10 minutes

Cooking time: 0 minute

Servings: 2

Ingredients:

1 large cucumber, peeled, seeded and chopped

1 large Granny Smith apple, peeled and chopped

1½ tablespoons of lime juice

1 tablespoon of mint leaves, chopped

2 teaspoons of raw honey, optional

Directions:

1. Blend all the ingredients in a blender.

2. Pour the mixture into ice cube trays and freeze.

3. Blend the frozen ice cubes into a slush and freeze in an airtight container.

Black Bean Brownies
Enjoy brownies without the extra calories.

Preparation time: 5 minutes

Cooking time: 18 minutes

Servings: 10-12

Ingredients:

1 15-ounce can of organic black beans, drained and rinsed thoroughly

½ cup of pure maple syrup

½ cup of chocolate chips

½ cup of quick oats

¼ cup of coconut oil

2 tablespoons of cocoa powder

2 teaspoon of alcohol-free pure vanilla extract

½ teaspoon of baking powder

¼ teaspoon of salt

Directions:

1. Preheat oven to 350°F.

2. Process all the ingredients except the chocolate chips in a food processor, until smooth. Add the chocolate chips and stir.

3. Pour the mixture into a prepared baking dish and bake for 18 minutes.

Avocado Chocolate Mousse
A treat to indulge in.

Preparation time: 3 hours 10 minutes

Cooking time: 5 minutes

Servings: 4

Ingredients:

4 over ripe avocados, peeled and pit removed

½ cup of agave

½ cup of bittersweet chocolate chips

½ cup of almond milk

1 tablespoon of pure vanilla extract

1/3 cup of almond milk

¼ teaspoon of fine salt

Fresh raspberries, garnish

Directions:

1. Melt the chips in a small bowl placed in saucepan of barely simmering water for about 3 minutes or until the chocolate is smooth and completely melted. Keep aside to cool a bit.

2. Process the melted chocolate and the remaining ingredients except the raspberries in a food processor until it is creamy and smooth.

3. Using a pastry bag, pipe or spoon the mixture into glasses and keep in the refrigerator for at least 3 hours.

4. Garnish with the raspberries and serve.

Lemon Cookies

Surprisingly easy to prepare.

Preparation time: 5 minutes

Cooking time: 8 hours

Servings: 12

Ingredients:

1 cup of unsweetened dried coconut

1 cup of cashews

3 tablespoons of lemon juice

1 tablespoon of maple syrup or agave nectar

Directions:

1. Process the cashews in a food processor until it looks like rough flour.

2. Add the dried coconut and continue processing until they are thoroughly combined.

3. Add the syrup and lemon. Process the mixture until it looks like dough.

4. Form the dough into cookies and allow to dehydrate for 8 hours.

Bliss Balls

If you aren't crazy about nuts, this is the dessert for you.

Preparation time: 15 minutes

Cooking time: 0 minute

Servings: 4-6

Ingredients:

6 medjool dates

½ cup of sunflower seeds

½ cup of dried apricots

½ cup of pumpkin seeds

¼ cup of raisins

1/3 cup of hemp seeds

½ teaspoon of ground cinnamon

¼ teaspoon of ground nutmeg

Directions:

1. Process all the ingredients in a food processor until it is smooth and comes together.

2. Form into balls and store in an airtight container in the refrigerator.

Ginger And Carrot Muffins

A fantastic dessert for everyone.

Preparation time: 10 minutes

Cooking time: 25 minutes

Servings: 12

Ingredients:

2 cups of almond flour

1½ cups of grated carrot

½ cup of unsweetened coconut, shredded

½ cup of melted macadamia nut oil or ghee

½ cup of toasted pecans, chopped

1/3 cup of maple syrup or 10 drops of stevia

3 eggs, whisked

1 teaspoon of baking soda

½ teaspoon of ground cloves

½ teaspoon of powdered ginger

Directions:

1. Preheat oven to 350°F.

2. In a large bowl, mix the flour, ginger, coconut, baking soda, and cloves together.

3. In a small bowl, mix the eggs, maple syrup and oil. Add this mixture to the flour mixture and combine thoroughly.

4. Pour the mixture into muffin pan and bake for 20-25 minutes or until the well cooked.

Almond Apricot Delight
Wholesome and nutritious.

Preparation time: 10 minutes

Cooking time: 0 minute

Servings: 2

Ingredients:

6½ ounces of low fat yogurt

1 cup of orange juice

5-6 fresh apricots

2-3 ice cubes

1 tablespoon of almonds, sliced

Grated nutmeg

Honey

Directions:

1. Blend all the ingredients except the nutmeg in a blender until it is thoroughly combined.

2. Sprinkle drink with the nutmeg and serve.

Banana Custard

No sugar added, yet very sweet.

Preparation time: 12 minutes

Cooking time: 40 minutes

Servings: 2

Ingredients:

9 fluid ounces of full fat coconut milk

4 eggs

2 medjool dates

2 over ripe bananas

1 teaspoon of almond essence

2 tablespoons of flaked almonds, optional

Directions:

1. Preheat oven to 350°F.

2. Blend all the ingredients except the almond flakes in a food processor or blender until it is thoroughly combined.

3. Grease 2 baking dishes and pour the mixture into them.

4. Bake for 40 minutes or until it is lightly golden and set.

5. Sprinkle with the almond flakes and serve.

Concluded!